Rafah ALMAMMOURI

The placenta and Gestational diabetes

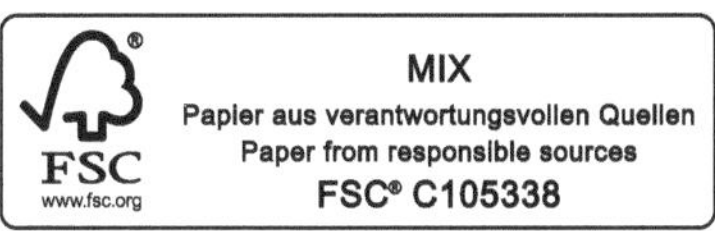

Printed by Books on Demand GmbH, Norderstedt / Germany

Rafah ALMAMMOURI

The placenta and Gestational diabetes

Placenta ,ubilical cord Dibetes

Noor Publishing

Imprint

Cover image: www.ingimage.com

Publisher:
Noor Publishing
is a trademark of
Dodo Books Indian Ocean Ltd. and OmniScriptum S.R.L publishing group

120 High Road, East Finchley, London, N2 9ED, United Kingdom
Str. Armeneasca 28/1, office 1, Chisinau MD-2012, Republic of Moldova, Europe
Printed at: see last page
ISBN: 978-620-5-63510-0

The placenta and Gestational diabetes

Prof.Dr.Rafah Hady Lateef
University of Babylon College of Science for Women

CONTENTS

Introduction:

The human haemochorial placenta is a complex and dynamic interface between embryonic and maternal tissues. It is an essential organ for fetal growth and development. It mounts adaptive responses to changes in the intrauterine environment, which occur during normal and also pathological pregnancies. (Gauster *et al.*,2012)

The placenta is formed as a result of the process of implantation, proliferation, and differentiation of the trophoblast; it is a vital organ for the survival, growth, and development of the embryo and fetus. The placenta measures approximately 20 cm in diameter, 2 to 3 cm thick, 500 g in weight, and is usually discoid in shape. The hormones of the placenta. (Prieto-Gómez *et al.,* 2018). The human placenta is composed of a fetal part or chorionic plate, and a maternal part or basal plate it is the synthesis of various hormones and growth factors, detoxification of maternal xenobiotics, immunologic barrier and dissipation of thermic energy resulting from foetal metabolism. the produce steroid hormones are human chrionic gonadotrophin(HCG), estrogens and progesterone, human chorionic somatomammotrophin (hcs), human placental growth hormone, human chrionic thyrotropin (hct), human chorionic adrenocorticotropin, insulin-like growth factor1(IGF-I), endothelial growth factor and relaxin).(Oratzs. 2014.)

Development of Placental Circulation start at twenty one day after coitus. Maternal and fetal circulation contributes to the development of placental circulation by vasculogenesis and angiogenesis. Upkeep of pregnancy requires both vasculogenesis and angiogenesis. Vasculogenesis is characterized by in situ differentiation of hemangiogenic stem cells derived from the pluripotent mesenchyme, followed by proliferation of angioblastic cells which give rise to precursor cells and followed by angiogenesis(Demir *et al.*,2006) . Significant blood flow in the feto–placental circulation at approximately 8weeks of gestation. (Clark *et al.*, 2015). The morphology of the umbilical cord is important. After about four weeks of gestation. It develops from the extra embryonic mesoderm and becomes the channel for blood vessels. The distance of the umbilical cord insertion from the placental center has been proposed as a clinically useful marker of placental insufficiency (Seema *et al.*,2019).

Fetal growth requires remodelling of maternal spiral arteries to provide an adequate maternal blood supply to the placenta. This arterial transformation is achieved by placental trophoblast cells, which invade into the uterine wall (Moffett *et al.*,2015). The angiogenic process is divided broadly into three major steps including the initiation of the angiogenic response, endothelial cell (EC) migration, proliferation and tube formation, and finally the maturation of the neovasculature. Angiogenesis is a complex, highly regulated process, involving the sprouting, splitting, and remodeling of the existing vessels.(Manisha *et al.*,2010). The DM2 affects most people with DM, characterized by a peripheral resistance to the action of insulin and a relative insulin deficiency which includes patients with DM1, DM2, and GDM, increases the possibility of complications during pregnancy and can cause adverse effects in the fetus. (GDM) is defined as abnormal or impaired glucose metabolism before pregnancy and it initially appears during pregnancy (Bastos & dos , 2015).

Kinase Domen Receptor (KDR) with subsequent over stimulation of endothelial cell migration. That this contributes to placental hypervascularization frequently observed in GDM pregnancies. (Felipe *et al.,* 2017).The immunohistochemistry detection Kit is a reliable and convenient tool to identify specified gene expression of VEGFA & R2 on tissues. VEGF is a major regulator of both physiological and pathological neovascularization so, considered as an important factor for the initiation of angiogenesis. (Khurri *et al.,*2010) The distribution of VEGF is observed in the placentas of women with GDM, and no VEGF is detected in the placental cellular compartments, which suggested a decrease in VEGF production. VEGF was always detected in the syncytiotrophoblast (ST) layer of term control tissues and term GDM tissues (Pietro *et al.*,2010),

The placentas from GDM are in a proangiogenic state characterized by hypervascularization frequently observed in GDM pregnancies. (Felipe *et al.*, 2017). Scanning electron microscopy is a standard method of biological investigation used for the explore cell surface. The scanning electron microscopy (SEM) can to demonstrate in a better aspect the morphological changes. (Castejon & Lopez

Human Placenta:

The placenta is a mirror that reflects the health of the fetus and continuously undergoes a change in weight, structure, shape and function in order to support the health of the fetus. vulnerable state. The placenta, as a fundamental organ within these complexities of intrauterine life, may represent an adaptive response and tries to compensate to prevent any foetal complications. (Mirbod P, 2018) It undergoes a change in weight, volume, structure, shape and functions continuously throughout gestation in order to support prenatal life. (Fahima *et al.*, 2011)

The placenta is an essential organ for fetal growth and development. It mounts adaptive responses to changes in the intrauterine environment, which occur during normal and also pathological pregnancies. (Gauster *et al.,*2012)

The most prevalent pathologies during pregnancy, such as hypertension, gestational diabetes mellitus (GDM), and intrauterine growth restriction (IUGR), can determine modifications in macro- and microscopic morphological features of the placenta and its free chorionic villi. In the fetus it may be accompanied by pathological manifestations, with the embryo's future quality of life, and even its viability, at risk(Ruth *et al.*,2018).

The placenta is formed as a result of the process of implantation, proliferation, and differentiation of the trophoblast; it is a vital organ for the survival, growth, and development of the embryo and fetus. The placenta measures approximately 20 cm in diameter, 2 to 3 cm thick, 500 g in weight, and is usually discoid in shape. The human placenta is composed of a fetal part or chorionic plate, and a maternal part or basal plate, each having well-defined features and functions. The chorionic plate is covered by the amnion. The amnion is made up of a single layer of stratified epithelium and amniotic mesenchyme, an avascular connective tissue. The placenta increases 14 g for every 100 g that the product increases. According to its weight, it is hypotrophic if less than 300 g and hypertrophic if more than 700 g. The umbilical cord is inserted in most cases in this part of the placenta in a slightly eccentric position, but there are other types of insertion such as marginal cord insertion, where the cord is attached to the side, or velamentous cord insertion, where the umbilical vessels are separated in the membranes at a certain distance from the placental margin, where they arrive surrounded only by a fold in the amnion. (Linda M, 2018).

The fetal vessels are unprotected in the placental membranes or umbilical cord (Wharton jelly), and can be bilobed or accessory .The basal plate represents the maternal surface of the placenta. It is an artificial surface that emerges from placental separation from the uterine wall during childbirth. The basal plate is a mixture of extravillous fetal trophoblasts and all types of maternal cells of the decidualized uterus, including decidual stromal cells, macrophages, and other immune cells. The basal plate also contains large amounts of extracellular matrix, fibrinoids, and blood clots. It is subdivided into elevated regions, called cotyledons. The cotyledons that are visible on the maternal surface of the placenta. (Carlson, 2014)

The placental cotyledons, also called lobules, develop from the joining of several chorionic villi. These cotyledons are separated by septa that derive from the basal decidua. A placenta will present a total of 20 to 35 cotyledons.(PRIETO *et al.*,2018).The placental villi are classified into stem villi, mature intermediate villi, terminal villi, immature intermediate villi and mesenchymal villi, based on the size of the villus, stromal characteristics and vessel structure . The syncytiotrophoblast is extremely attenuated and covers the terminal villi forming the maternal-fetal exchange surface. (Burton, 2006)

The first component of the embryo is the trophoblast, from which the placenta originates after implantation, the extraembryonic mesoderm appears, located between the trophoblast and the blastocyst cavity thus, the trophoblast and the extraembryonic mesoderm will constitute a common structure, the chorion this is a tissue from which the villi will form that will absorb nutrients and oxygen from the maternal blood to then be transported to what will be the body of the embryo. (Carlson, 2014)

These villi will first be composed, externally, of syncytiotrophoblast and a cytotrophoblast nucleus, and will receive the number of primary chorionic villi then, the extraembryonic mesoderm arises from the nucleus of the primary villi, at which point they become known as secondary villi. Finally, small embryonic blood vessels appear in the extraembryonic mesoderm, and there the villi begin to be called tertiary. With respect to the extension of the villi, they can be defined as “free” when they extend from the villous stem and have no fixation in the cytotrophoblastic shell, floating in the blood chamber bathed in maternal blood. Therefore, the so-called "anchoring villi" are those that reach the cytotrophoblast envelope, and through this reach the decidua, thereby ensuring fixation of the embryo. (Roa *et al.,* 2012).

The blastocyst is surrounded by trophoblast and thus everything will tend to the formation of chorionic villi; however, the trophoblast from which the implantation began can grow further, causing greater branching of its chorionic villi this region of the chorion is called the "chorion frondosum", corresponding then to the embryonic portion of the placenta. Therefore, the mature placental barrier will comprise the following components: syncytiotrophoblast, cytotrophoblast, extraembryonic mesoderm, and the endothelial lining of the chorionic vessels (Prieto *et al.*, 2011).

The maturity of the chorionic villi can be evaluated by development they reach on the villous tree in relation to the gestational age determined by clinical history or by the weight of the newborn and the placenta. During normal gestation there may be disruptions in the maturation process of the placental villi, accelerating or delaying it in a normal mature placenta, immature intermediate villi can be found in the central portion of the placentoma or placental lobule these are villi that continue with their proliferation and represent a type of growth reserve in addition, during pregnancy, the chorionic villi can present degenerative changes that, within certain parameters, can be considered normal. However, when the villi begin to appear compromised in large proportion, this can affect the normal development of the fetus, causing structural malformations the lack of placental development can directly bring about congenital defects, and villous lesions such as trophoblastic necrosis, edema, immaturity, thrombosis, and trophoblast inclusions are also found more frequently in neural tube defects and chromosomal disorders (Castejón and Molinaro, 2004)

The functions of the placenta are of great importance for the fetus and the mother. First of all, the exchange of metabolic and gaseous products between mother and fetus, acting as a barrier between maternal and fetal circulation this is where the synthesis of substances, such as cholesterol, fatty acids, and glycogen are produced, and an immune function, permitting the transmission of antibodies from mother to fetus. The placenta is the bidirectional mother-fetus/fetus-mother transport through diffusion. Many substances, such as oxygen, water, hormones, electrolytes, drugs, and toxic elements, pass from maternal circulation to the fetal blood (Carlson, 2014).

Transport of oxygen, water, and electrolytes. It must be considered relevant that the passage of glucose to the fetus by diffusion is its main source of energy. Free fatty acids also cross the placental barrier and are then esterified in the fetus to form triglycerides amino acids can also pass through the placental barrier, thus managing to satisfy the needs of the fetus in terms of protein synthesis transport of hormones and antibodies. Steroid hormones cross the placental barrier freely protein and peptide hormones cannot cross the placental barrier; antibodies are one exception among elements of a protein nature transport of drugs and toxic substances. Most drugs, toxic substances, and their metabolic products cross the placental barrier. (Prieto *et al.,* 2018).

Structure of the Placenta:

Placenta is a combination of tissues of embryo and mother, carrying the exchange of substances. It consists of amniotic membrane, chorion frondosum and decidua's Placental development starts with the implantation of the blastocyst into the endometrial surface. Subsequently, the placental structure continuously develops by a series of differentiation and proliferation processes of trophoblast cells that eventually lead to placental villi of varying degree of maturation. (Sun *et al*., 2013)

During implantation and subsequent placentation in the human, populations of trophoblast cells invade the endometrium and maternal vasculature within the uterus. On reaching the spiral arteries within the myometrium, trophoblast invasiveness stops. (Kaufmann and Burton,1994)

It is the fastes growing organ of human body. The placenta grows from a single cell to 5×1010 cells in 38 week the fetus, placenta and mother form a triad of equilibrium the maternal blood is supplied to the placenta by spiral arteries (100-150) are formed and 50-200 veins. The normal placenta parenchyma is divided into 10-40 lobes by septa chorionic plate 60-70 fetal stem vessels supplies a villous tree. During the first twelve week of development the placenta consist of mesenchymal villi after this period subsequently stem villi, immature intermediate, mature intermediate, mature intermediate and terminal villi are formed the terminal villi can be recognized by the presence of syncytio-vascular membranes the development of this membranes in the third trimester is provide the fetus with adequate amount of oxygen by diffusion is highly dependent upon the distance between maternal and fetal blood. (Carlson,2014)

Villus capillaries that lie below syncytiotrophoplast directly opposite to the vessel wall. Immature intermediate villi can recognized by fine reticular connective tissue with Hofbaure cells. After 12 week immature intermediate villi are formed that disappeared after 24 week of pregnancy. In a mature placenta the main the anchoring or stem villus is connected with the chorionic plate and consist of dense fibrous tissue with large arteries and veins with a clearly recognizable muscular layer. The trophoblast lining of the stem villi is slowly replaced by fibrin during development. Mature intermediate villi are the connection between the stem villi and the terminal villi. The terminal villi can be recognized from 30-32 weeks, 40% of the placental villi consist of these terminal villi. (Saddler, 2004)

The chorionic villi constitute the major fetal component of the placenta. They consist of a mesenchymal core containing matrix, cells and fetal blood vessels. During the first trimester the villi are covered by the two-layered epithelium of trophoblast including the cellular, non-invasive, villous cytotrophoblast and an outer layer of multinucleated syncytiotrophoblast, which is bathed in maternal blood. As gestation continues the cytotrophoblast becomes discontinuous and the syncytiotrophoblast thinner. Nutrients from the maternal blood are transported across these compartments to reach the fetal vessels. Some of the chorionic villi are free, other villi attached to the decidua at the site of invasion forming the anchoring villi. At these sites villous cytotrophoblast cells proliferate and break through the syncytiotrophoblast to form cytotrophoblast columns and invade the decidua basalis. Some of these extravillous cytotrophoblast cells also invade the uterine spiral arteries, becoming endovascular trophoblast, partly replacing the endothelial cells. These cells seem to augment the vessel walls. (Guodong *et al.,* 2013)

The placenta is a foetal organ situated between mother and fetus. In addition to serving as a channel for maternal fuels destined to nourish the growing fetus it fulfils a wide spectrum of other functions including the synthesis of various hormones and growth factors, detoxification of maternal xenobiotics, immunologic barrier and thermic energy resulting from fetal metabolism. Maternal diabetes is associated with concentration changes of various hormones, cytokines and metabolites in the maternal as well as fetal circulation. In addition to differential effects of the diabetic environment of mother and fetus, the distinct processes affected by maternal diabetes also critically depend on the time period in gestation when the diabetic insult occurs (Desoye and Hauguel, 2007)

Most villi freely float in the intervillous space at the tips of some villi cytotrophoblasts accumulate and invade into the decidua. These villi physically anchor the placenta and, later, the foetus in the maternal endometrium, and are formed mainly in the first trimester of pregnancy as a result of proliferation, differentiation and invasion of trophoblasts. A proportion of invasive extravillous cytotrophoblasts also invades the endometrial spiral arteries and remodels them into low resistance arteries. This increases the utero-placental blood flow into the intervillous space, thus ensuring adequate maternal nutrient supply to the foetus. Since placental anchoring and establishment of maternal blood supply are key processes in placental development, their dysregulation is associated with pregnancy diseases: Shallow invasion has been implicated in intra-uterine growth restriction (IUGR). (Kaufmann *et al.,*2003)

Placental cells at the maternal–fetal interface, Cytotrophoblasts are mononucleated cells that proliferate and undergo fusion and biochemical differentiation to originate the syncytiotrophoblast. The syncytiotrophoblast is a multinucleated cell layer devoid of proliferative activity, which is in intimate contact with the maternal blood. The cytotrophoblasts may also acquire invasive capacity, invading maternal decidua (decidual cell) and part of the myometrium (smooth muscle cell), blood vessels, and uterine glands forming the interstitial extravillous trophoblast, endovascular extravillous trophoblasts, and endoglandular extravillous trophoblasts respectively. Endovascular extravillous trophoblasts replace the endothelial cells of spiral artery, leading to the widening of artery lumen, which decreases the resistance against blood flow that irrigates the fetus . Interstitial extravillous trophoblast fuse and form the multinucleated giant trophoblast cells, which are unable to further invade the uterine tissues. (Mariana, 2016)

It is one components of human placenta. It is a non fibrous, a cellular, homogenous material derived from cellular secretion and cellular degeneration. Fibriniod is composed of two types that differ in their origin and composition. Fibrin type fibrinoid is derived from the coagulation cascade is composed of fibrin. The function of fibrin support of the stem villi, regulation of intervillous circulation by clotting of poorly perfused areas, barrier to trophoblastic invasion. Matrix- type fibrinoid is a secretory product of extravillous trophoblastic cells is composed of collagen ιv and glycoprotein of the extracellular matrix. Intravillous deposition of fibrinoid is increased in pregnancies associated with GDM. The deposits begin as small nodules that grow to replace the stroma of villi. Fibrinoid is may occur secondary to an immunological attack against the villous cytotrophoblast, clotting of blood and may be due to villous degeneration (Rebecca, 2005)

Function of fibrin includes mechanical stability to support of chorionic plate, basal plat and stem villi. Regulation of intervillous circulation by clotting of poorly perfused areas. Barrier to trophoplastic invation. Alternative route of maternofetal after damage to syncytiotrophoblastic surfaces. Function of fibriniod includes adhesiveness of the placenta to the uterine wall, assistance with reepitheliazation of damaged villous surfaces immunoprotection to mask fetal antigens, acts as an immune absorptive sponge and promotion of trophoblastic invasion. (Arsenio *et al.*,2019)

Function of Placenta:

The placenta is essential for fetal growth and development. It serving as a channel for maternal fuels destined to nourish the growing fetus, it is the synthesis of various hormones and growth factors, detoxification of maternal xenobiotics, immunologic barrier and dissipation of thermic energy resulting from foetal metabolism. The placenta is exposed to regulatory influences of mother and foetus although at different surfaces as the microvillous syncytiotrophoblast membrane as well as the basal syncytiotrophoblast membrane and the endothelial cells. (Desoye *et al.*,2007) The placental Transport contributes to insulin resistance during pregnancy via its secretion of hormones and cytokines. As the barrier between the maternal and fetal environments, the placenta itself is also exposed to hyperglycemia and its consequences during GDM. This can impact transport of glucose, amino acids, and lipids across the placenta: Glucose is the primary energy source for the fetus and the placenta, and therefore must be readily available at all times. For this reason, insulin is not required for the placental transport of glucose. The receptivity of the placenta to glucose uptake means sensitive to maternal hyperglycemia, due to fetal growth and macrosomia. (Zhang et al.,2016) .

placental hormones

The release of placental hormones into maternal circulation has been the target as biomarkers diagnosing pregnancy related diseases. The study of hormone production by human placenta and the function of each hormone in different pregnancy events represent a test. Human placental explants or isolated primary human cytotrophoblasts are used to assess the endocrine function of human placenta.. the cytotrophoblast, have the main characteristics of human cytotrophoblast cells, including the synthesis of placental hormones, e.g. human chorionic gonadotrophin (HCG), progesterone, oestrogens . (Panelk *et al.,* 2011).

During pregnancy, the pregnant must adapt her body systems to support nutrient and oxygen supply for growth of the fetus in utero . Failure to suitably adjust maternal physiology to the mother state may result in pregnancy complications, including GDM and abnormal birth weight. The placenta, which forms the functional border separating the maternal and fetal circulations, is significant for mediating adaptations in maternal physiology. (Tina *et al* ., 2018)

Pregnancy is a physiological state characterized by radical changes in the hormonal profile. In fact, during this period, placenta synthesis and secretes several hormones that are crucial for the regulation of distinct pregnancy stages, such as decidualization and implantation and labour, and also for the maternal metabolic adaptation and preparation for breastfeeding., altered levels of placenta hormones are associated with poor gestational outcome. The deficient production of these hormones may also contribute to the altered placental development observed in these conditions. In this way, the combination of measurements of different hormones, analysed with other clinical examinations and risk factors, in attempting to find reliable biomarkers. (Carlson, 2014) The exchange function allows placenta act as an excretory, a respiratory, a nutritive, a protective organ to the fact that the placental barrier can prevent passage of most of the organisms to the fetal blood,, it allows the passage of antibodies mainly IgG to protect the baby even after delivery. placental hormone synthesis: the syncytiotrophoblasts are an endocrine organ during pregnancy, the produce steroid hormones are human chrionic gonadotrophin(HCG), estrogens and progesterone, human chorionic somatomammotrophin (hcs), human placental growth hormone, human chrionic thyrotropin (hct), human chorionic adrenocorticotropin, insulin-like growth factor1(IGF-I), endothelial growth factor, hPL human placental lactogen (hpL) and relaxin).(Saddler ,1995)

The endocrine function of the human placenta is critical for the success of distinct pregnancy events , these endocrine alterations may be helpful in predicting and diagnosing pregnancy-related conditions, providing an early planning of the best clinical strategies to manage these conditions. A large amount of evidence exists supporting the role of estradiol, progesterone, hPL in the initiation and extension of hyperphagia, hyperlipidemia, hyperinsulinemia, and insulin resistance. The peptide hormones hCG have a minor role in these changes. (Mariana., 2016)

Intrauterine tissues (placenta, amnion, chorion, decidua) express hormones that play a decisive role in maternal-fetal physiological interactions. The excessive or deficient release of some placental hormones in association with gestational diseases may reflect an abnormal differentiation of the placenta, an impaired fetal metabolism, or an adaptive response of the feto-placental unit to adverse conditions.(Reis *et al.*, 2002).

In syncytiotrophoblast is an endocrine tissue that synthesizes important steroid and protein hormones during the greater part of gestation. particular, the Hormones produced by the placenta include human chorionic gonadotropin, chorionic somatomammotropin, or placental lactogen, whose action stimulates changes in the metabolism of carbohydrates in the mother in relation to the nutrition of the fetus. For example, inhibiting maternal insulin and leading to an elevation in glycemia levels, thus favoring the passage of glucose to the fetus. Progesterone, estrogens, and relaxin are also produced in the placenta.(P RIETO., 2018)

The major factors contributing to GDM are the placental hormones, such as human placental lactogen, progesterone, growth hormone and prolactin. These hormones cause the decreased phosphorylation of insulin receptor substrate-1 (IRS-1), resulting in thorough insulin resistance . As reported 50 % of beta cell function in a normal pregnancy , and to maintain euglycemia, the pancreas should compensate by increasing insulin secretion by 2–2.5 times.(Cianni *et al.,* 2003)

Placental blood Circulation

Development of Placental Circulation start at twenty one day after coitus. Maternal and fetal circulation contributes to the development of placental circulation by vasculogenesis and angiogenesis.Upkeep of pregnancy requires both vasculogenesis and angiogenesis. Vasculogenesis is characterized by in situ differentiation of hemangiogenic stem cells derived from the pluripotent mesenchyme, followed by proliferation of angioblastic cells which give rise to precursor cells. This is followed by angiogenesis. (Demir *et al.,* 2006)

The chorionic plate contains the vessels that continue with those of the umbilical cord. Derived from the two umbilical arteries, The chorionic veins give rise to the single umbilical vein. the chorionic arteries present a centrifugal distribution pattern in their terminal branches that allow them to supply blood to the villi. The chorionic veins are direct continuations of the veins of the villous trees (stem villi, attached to the plate that reaches the cotyledon) and usually crosses underneath to the chorionic arteries. (Prieto Gómez *et al.*, 2008). The vascular pattern of chorionic blood vessels of placenta is described as of two types- Magistral and dispersal).In the dispersal pattern umbilical vessels undergo successive divisions and rapidly diminish in caliber while in magistral pattern umbilical vessels give side branches and the caliber of vessels is almost equal up to periphery.The vascular character of foetal placental vasculature is already recognizable at 12th week of pregnancy. (Yousuf *et al.*, 2010) Figure2.2.

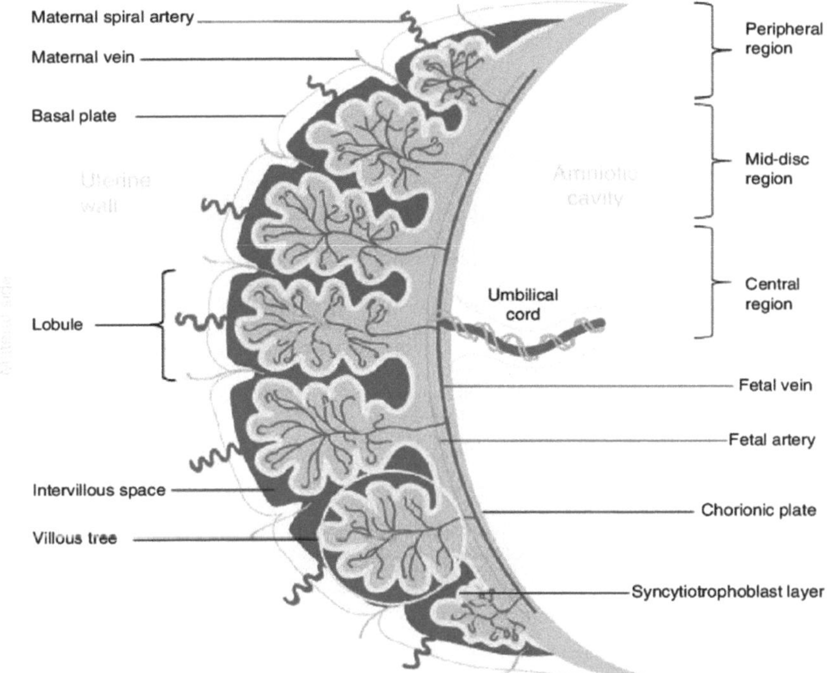

Figure2.2 Blood circulation of placenta (Rani et al., 2016)

Significant blood flow in the feto–placental circulation at approximately eight weeks of gestation, Umbilical cord contain two umbilical arteries and one vein. The two umbilical arteries transport the fetal blood to the placenta, and then they branch off in the chorionic plate, thus creating networks of capillaries in the chorionic villi. The largest placental blood vessels (termed the chorionic vessels). The arteries at the umbilical cord insertion point measure up to 5 mm in diameter. In normal placentas, they branch in a mostly dichotomous manner to ultimately form approximately 60–100 chorionic arteries as small as 0.8 mm in diameter that branch into villous tissue.The villous trees contain the placental villous blood vessels, which follow the branching structure of the villous trees for several generations before pending the capillary structures which fill the distal trimmings of the villous trees. Fetoplacental vessels are found in chorionic villi bathed in maternal blood and this close proximity permits efficient exchange of solutes and gases between the maternal and fetal circulations without intermingling of the two. (Carlson,2014)

The arrangement allows the development, growth, and remodeling of fetoplacental vessels to be matched to the fetal need while rendering them vulnerable to changes on both the maternal and fetal sides. As these vessels extend into the underlying villus tree, they branch further into multiple arterioles and venules that end in a dense network of capillary ‘convolutes. Maternal spiral arteries credit oxygenated blood and nutrients into the intervillus space. (Rani et al., 2016) The space is a hollow expanse, into which the villous trees from the fetal circulation extend. The intervillus space is bounded on the maternal side by the basal plate, and on the fetal side by the chorionic plate. The villous trees and terminal villi contain the terminal umbilical arterioles and capillaries that arise from the umbilical arteries and transport the deoxygenated blood and waste products from the fetus for exchange in the intervillus space. These vessels return blood to the fetus via the umbilical veins. Clark *et al.,* (2015)

At the end of the pregnancy and each of placental lobule will present from 1 to 4 stem villi. Approximately 150 mL of maternal blood per minute is exchanged between the decidua and the villi, so that the uterine spiral arteries carry maternal blood (oxygenated and with nutrients) to the villi, diffusing the components transported by the blood through the placental barrier and reaching the chorionic vessels, where the return blood will circulate to the embryo. Similarly, the transport of waste and carbon dioxide occurs, but from the chorionic vessels, diffusing to the maternal blood located outside the villi. The exchange occurs in this sector and then the capillaries become blood vessels, which continue them, enlarging until they form the umbilical vein. (P Rieto., 2018)

The umbilical vein is the one responsible for delivering oxygenated blood to the fetus, and it also contains nutrients and other substances that it receives from the maternal blood, whereas the blood with carbon dioxide and the waste pass through the umbilical arteries.The maternal blood arrives at a type of pool not contained in blood vessels.Between 80 and 100 spiral arteries of the endometrium spill their contents into the intervillous spaces and bathe the villi.This blood arrives at the villi with low pressure, but it manages to reach the villi. The route of the blood follows the villi until arriving at the capillary networks of the fetal vessels, so that the previously mentioned exchange of substances occurs.The exchange of metabolic and gaseous products between mother and fetus, acting as a barrier between maternal and fetal circulation. This is where the synthesis of substances, such as cholesterol, fatty acids, and glycogen are produced, in addition to an immune function, permitting the transmission of antibodies from mother to fetus. (Mariana., 2016)

The most notable function of the placenta is the bidirectional mother-fetus/fetus-mother transport through different transport mechanisms, such as simple diffusion, facilitated diffusion and active transport using adenosine triphosphate. Many substances, such as oxygen, water, hormones, electrolytes, drugs, and toxic elements, pass from maternal circulation to the fetal blood. Fetoplacental vessels are found in chorionic villi bathed in maternal blood and this close proximity permits efficient exchange of solutes and gases between the maternal and fetal circulations without intermingling of the two.The arrangement allows the development, growth, and remodeling of fetoplacental vessels to be matched to the fetal need while rendering them vulnerable to changes on both the maternal and fetal sides. (Carlson, 2014).

Remodeling of Spiral Artery

Fetal growth requires remodelling of maternal spiral arteries to provide an adequate maternal blood supply to the placenta.This arterial transformation is achieved by placental trophoblast cells, which invade into the uterine wall. Fetal growth restriction is associated with reduced remodelling of maternal spiral arteries by trophoblast cells.In normal pregnancy, extravillous trophoblast cells migrate as far as the myometrium and also infiltrate into the arterial media and endothelium of maternal spiral arteries. This results in dilatation and increased flow of maternal blood at low pressure into the intervillous space.In pregnancies affected by gestational complication , the depth of trophoblast invasion is reduced with less spiral artery remodelling. Blood flows at higher pressure and is more pulsatile, resulting in placental stress, reduced placental development and poor fetal growth.Under-invasion is associated with fetal growth restriction; but if invasion is excessive large babies can result. (Moffett *et al.*, 2015)

Fetal growth in utero depends on the development of a good maternal blood supply to the placenta that requires modification of the uterine spiral arteries.Trophoblast cells from the placenta invade deeply into the stroma to effect arterial conversion.The extravillous trophoblast cells (EVT) encircle the arteries, and then cause direct destruction of the smooth muscle of the arterial wall with complete loss of vasoconstriction.(figure 2.3) Trophoblast cells only move down the inside of the arteries to replace the endothelium and functionally modify the media. (Parham & Moffett,2013)

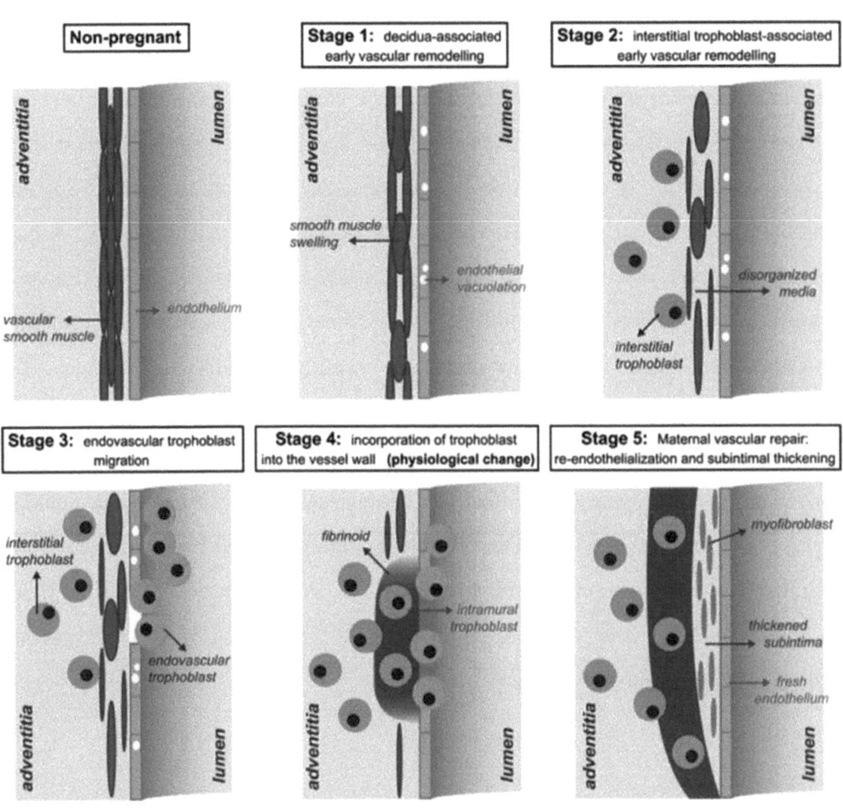

Figure 2.3 Vascular remodeling of spiral artery. (Saunders .2009)

Early remodeling partly depends on the presence of Interstitial trophoplast .During early pregnancy, the spiral arteries undergo extensive remodeling. This remodeling is driven by extravillous trophoblast cells as well as by Uterine Natural Killer Cells (uNKs). uNKs are evolutionarily preserved, having been shown to accumulate in the uterus during pregnancy in human. Interstitial trophoplast-associated remodeling should be interrupted, preceding the endovascular trophoblast-associated remodelling. (Mariana., 2016)

Trophoblast plays an important role in the complete physiological change of the spiral arteries. In the first place the earliest, decidua-associated alteration. This is vital for making a clear distinction between decidua and trophoblast-include remodeling. These early changes with increasing blood flow endovascular verses interstitial trophoplast invasion. In early pregnancy spiral arteries become surrounded by interstitial trophoblast. The earliest stage in vascular remodeling consist of endothelial vacuolation and some swelling in individual muscle cells. Invasion of stromal and perivascular tissue by interstitial trophoblast is associated with further disorganization of the vascular smooth muscle layer. (figure 2.4).Trophoblast becomes embedded intramurally within a fibrinoid-layer, which replaces the original vascular smooth muscle. Finally reendothelialization occurs, containing α-actin immunopositive myointimal cells.(Pijnenborg *et.al.,* 2006) Extensive vascular remodeling and stabilization of the vascular bed occur in second half of gestation. (Mayhew, 2002)

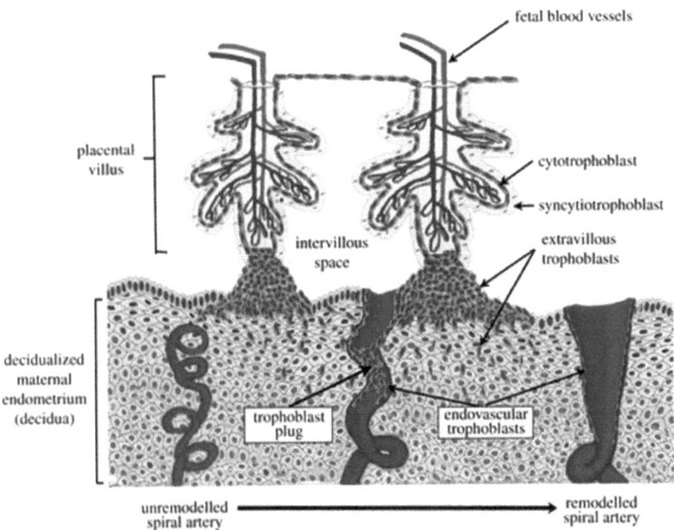

Figure 2.(4) Maternal blood supply to establishment of placenta.(Saghian *et al.*, 2019)

During implantation and subsequent placentation in the human, populations of trophoblast cells invade the endometrium and maternal vasculature within the uterus. On reaching the spiral arteries within the myometrium, trophoblast invasiveness ceases (Sandra *et al.*, 2000).

The trophoblasts is epithelial cells have different phenotypes and form the in chorionic villi, finger-shaped structures. Cytotrophoblasts are mononucleated cells that are able to proliferate and differentiate into other trophoblast.com subtypes, functioning as a precursor for the syncytiotrophoblast and extravillous trophoblasts (EVT). cytotrophoblasts fuse and undergo biochemical differentiation, giving rise to the multinucleated syncytiotrophoblast. The syncytial layer has no proliferative capacity and is in intimate contact with maternal blood, participating in fetal nourishment, gas exchange and also playing important roles in other placental functions, mainly in protein biosynthesis. .(Mariana , 2016)

Cytotrophoblasts may also acquire invasive properties, forming the EVT. These trophoblasts are able to invade and remodel maternal tissues (interstitial EVT) and uterine spiral artery (endovascular EVT), leading to the widening of artery lumen, reducing the resistance against blood flow that irrigates the fetus. EVT may also invade and remodel uterine glands (endoglandular EVT), which is important to provide nutrition to the embryo. Trophoblast subtypes interact with each other and with decidual cells, Hofbaüer cells, endothelial cells, vascular smooth muscle cells, providing a sole microenvironment that is vital for pregnancy outcome and fetal development. The hormones produced by EVT contribute to vascular and uterine tissue remodelling and to regulate EVT migration and invasion (Jia *et al.*, 2013).

Villous cytotrophoblast cells proliferate and break through the syncytiotrophoblast to form cytotrophoblast columns and invade the decidua basalis. Some of these extravillous cytotrophoblast cells also invade the uterine spiral arteries, becoming endovascular trophoblast, partly replacing the endothelial cells. Cytotrophoblasts are mononucleated cells that proliferate and undergo fusion and biochemical differentiation to originate the syncytiotrophoblast. The cytotrophoblasts may also acquire invasive capacity, invading maternal decidua (decidual cell) and part of the myometrium (smooth muscle cell), blood vessels, and uterine glands forming the interstitial extravillous trophoblast, endovascular extravillous trophoblasts, and endoglandular extravillous trophoblasts respectively. Endovascular extravillous trophoblasts replace the endothelial cells of spiral artery, leading to the widening of artery lumen, which decreases the resistance against blood flow that irrigates the fetus . Interstitial extravillous trophoblast fuse and form the multinucleated giant trophoblast cells, which are unable to further invade the uterine tissues. .(Saghian *et al.*,2019)

The fibrinolytic system plays a role in several physiological and pathophysiological processes, such as hemostatic balance, tissue remodeling, angiogenesis and reproduction. Normal pregnancy is a state of hypercoagulability. Fibrinolytic system is depressed during pregnancy. the major inhibitor of the fibrinolytic system: plasminogen activator inhibitor type 1 (PAI-1). PAI-1 is responsible for 60% of the PA-inhibitory activity in the plasma. (Yao Ye *et al.*,2017).

PAI-1 Inhibits Trophoblast Invasion. Trophoblast invasion at the maternal-fetal interface is a key process during implantation and placentation, and during this process extravillous cytotrophoblasts (EVT) acquire invasive properties, which are able to invade and remodel maternal tissues (interstitial EVT) and uterine spiral artery (endovascular EVT). EVT can degrade extracellular matrix (ECM) to promote cell migration to the maternal side. EVT invasion in early pregnancy occurs in a relatively low-oxygen (3%) environment, which is mediated by a general inhibition of the plasminogen activator system, as well as many adhesion molecules, growth factors, cytokines, interleukins, ECM components, and various placental hormones. (Silva & Serakides,2016)

2.1.6 Angiogenesis

The angiogenic process is divided broadly into three major steps including the initiation of the angiogenic response, endothelial cell (EC) migration, proliferation and tube formation, and finally the maturation of the neovasculature. Angiogenesis is a complex, highly regulated process, involving the sprouting, splitting, and remodeling of the existing vessels.(Manisha *et al.,* 2010),.

placental angiogenesis, also the mean number of redundant capillary connections per terminal villus and the incidence of vascular hyperplasia (chorioangiosis) . Madazli *et al.*, 2008)

Angiogenesis, defined as the process of forming new blood vessels that arise from preexisting ones, is essential to fetal growth and normal placental development. Generally, there are two phases in angiogenesis: branching angiogenesis with the formation of looped capillaries, and nonbranching angiogenesis with the formation of longer capillaries.(Blackburn, 2013) .

Vasculogenesis is characterized by in situ differentiation of hemangiogenic stem cells derived from the pluripotent mesenchyme, followed by proliferation of angioblastic cells which give rise to precursor cells. This is followed by angiogenesis. (Demir *et al.*,2004)
The process of angiogenesis involves proliferation, migration, and maturation of both maternal and fetal endothelial cells (Kingdom *et al.*,2009

Placental angiogenesis one of the main steps in the placenta formation is the development of its highly structured and specialized net of blood vessels. Formation of placental blood vessels occurs with (i) vasculogenesis, which begins at the end of the third week of gestation and corresponds to the formation of the first vascular plexus from pluripotent progenitor cells which then differentiate into endothelial cells, and (ii) angiogenesis, which begins at the end of the fourth week of gestation and where the first vascular plexus are expanded and remodeled. (Gutiérrez *et al.*, 2016)

Meanwhile expression of angiogenic factors as well as the angiogenic process itself are under regulation by glycaemia, insulin, and hypoxia. (Chen and Zheng, 2014 ;) This process is finely tuned and regulated by different angiogenic factors including the vascular endothelial growth factor (VEGF), placental growth factor (PlGF), angiopoietins , fibroblast growth factor 2 (FGF2), and the insulin/insulin-like growth factors (INS/IGF) system Jauniaux, *et al* . (2000)

Expression of these factors is highly regulated throughout gestation and is mainly attributed to trophoblast cells, Hofbauer cells, and smooth muscle cells, Since expression of angiogenic factors as well as the angiogenic process itself are under regulation by glycaemia, insulin, and hypoxia Chen and Zheng (2014) , vasculogenesis and angiogenesis processes at the fetoplacental vasculature are susceptible to alterations by a diabetic environment, such as in GDM or pregestational diabetes mellitus. Besides activation of the angiogenic factors, activation of ERS and pathways and dyslipidaemia (Oh *et al.,* 2016)

Angiogenesis in DMT1 and DMT2 affect the entire process vasculogenesis and angiogenesis while GDM seems to impact the microvascular remodeling at angiogenesis(Jarmuzek *et al.*,(201 5 .

At 3rd trimester of pregnancy, the effect of DMT1, DMT2, and GDM on these phenomena is similar resulting in increased branching and surface area of villous capillaries Jirkovská *et al.,* (2002). Since GDM associates with developing longer umbilical cords compared with normal pregnancies Georgiadis *et al.,* 2014) it is suggested that placental hypervascularization in diabetes mellitus is mainly attributed to increased angiogenesis(Leach, 2011)

The later is partially explained by a placental hypoxia condition resulting from the fetal hyperglycaemia in diabetes mellitus. Fetal hyperglycaemia triggers fetal hyperinsulinemia, over-activating fetal metabolism leading to increased oxygen demand Jarmuzek *et al* .(2015),.fetal hypoxia promotes the expression of angiogenic factors during the physiological placental angiogenesis at the 1st trimester of pregnancy when the oxygen level is reduced since the level of Fibroblast growth factor-2 (FGF-2) is also regulated by hypoxia. (Seo *et al.,* 2013)

Increased in both the placenta and umbilical cord blood in diabetic pregnancies this growth factor emerges as a candidate to explain the hypervascularization in placentas from diabetes mellitus. Knowing that insulin is an angiogenic factor in endothelial cells fetal hyperinsulinemia would have profound effects on placental and fetal vascular changes associated with maternal diabetes mellitus in pregnancy (Lassance *et al* 2013) ,.

VEGF expression was shown to be lower in human placentas likely due to increased expression Thus, responses of endoplasmic reticulum stress (ERS) to a stressor will also result in an altered synthes.(Jarmuzek *et. al*,. 2015) is and/or release of proangiogenic factors in the human placenta vascular bed. (Aditiawarman, 2014) .In addition to placental angiogenesis, also the mean number of jobless capillary connections per terminal villus and the incidence of vascular hyperplasia (chorioangiosis) .(Madazli *et.al.,2008).* A hallmark of GDM is increased villous immaturity and increased measures of angiogenesis.(Huynh *et al*., 2015)

Umbilical cord

The morphology of the umbilical cord is important It can provide more clinically useful information about the placental state. After about four weeks of gestation. It develops from the extra embryonic mesoderm and becomes the channel for blood vessels. It is composed of two arteries and one vein to maintain the feto-maternal exchange of oxygen, nutrients and waste products. These blood vessels are surrounded with wharton's jelly (is mainly amucopolysaccharides) a gelatinous stroma and covered by a single layer of amnion to provide flexibility, mobility and strength to resist compression and the fetus to move freely .Umbilical cord lacks vasa vasorum and depends on the blood in the umbilical vessels and wharton's jelly for its nutrition. Diabetes exerts a heavy toll on the vascular system. Vessels of all sizes are affected from aorta down to the smallest arterioles and capillaries. Maternal diabetes significantly influences the expression of genes in the umbilical cord and alters the umbilical vessel phenotype, with possible long term consequences for the neonate. GDM causes rupture of endothelium of umbilical arteries, unduly dilated umbilical vein, disruption and degeneration of muscle fibers and empty spaces in the wharton's jelly. (Seema *et al.,* 2019) and (Kulkarni *et al.,* 2007)

Umbilical cord insertion

Umbilical cord insertion into the placenta is varied. The distance of the umbilical cord insertion from the placental center has been proposed as a clinically useful marker of placental insufficiency. Marginal velamentous and furcated are rare and associated with pathology. Marginal and velamentous insertions are suggested to result from disturbances of implantation.The umbilical cord insertion was considered velamentous when it was located in the membranes, furcated when there was split in umbilical vessels and left wharton's jelly before reaching the chorionic plate surface, marginal when the distance between the cord insertion and the placental margin was less than 1 cm and central when the cord is placed at the centre and 1 cm away from the centre and the remaining were called eccentric. Coiling index is probably one of the most frequently reported umbilical cord related parameters in high risk pregnancies. Pre-eclampsia and gestational diabetes have been suggested as maternal risk factors for abnormal coiling. (Seema *et al*., 2019)

Diabetes Mellitus:

Diabetes mellitus is recognized as being a syndrome, a collection of disorders that have hyperglycaemia and glucose intolerance as their hallmark, due either to insulin deficiency or to the impaired effectiveness of insulin's action, or to a combination of these. Diabetes is the disease or disorder of pancreas by which pancreas stop the secretion of insulin in the body. Insulin allow the glucose enter in to the cells which provide energy to every cells of the body without insulin, glucose can not enter in to the cell. Those part which help to secrete insulin, the part which are defective which is known as diabetes type 1. In the type of diabetes mellitus the overall diabetes cases 10%. The type-1 diabetes which is most occurring in children. About 90% of incidence of type-2 diabetes mellitus. It is mainly occurring after the age 40s. In this case insulin secreted but only in low amount and it is co-related of our life style such as overeating, physical activity. (Manish *et al.*, 2019).

Classification of diabetes mellitus

Two major forms of diabetes are recognized in Western countries; insulin dependent diabetes mellitus (IDDM, type I diabetes) and non-insulin dependant diabetes (NIDDM, type II diabetes).

1 Insulin dependent diabetes mellitus (IDDM)

The subclass of diabetes, type I diabetes, is generally characterized by the abrupt onset of severe symptoms, dependence on exogenous insulin to sustain life caused by absolute insulin deficiency. IDDM is the most prevalent type of diabetes among children and young adults in developing countries. It is a catabolic disorder in which circulating insulin is virtually absent, plasma glucagon is elevated, and the pancreatic B cells fail to respond to all insulinogenic stimuli .Type I diabetes is thought to result from an infectious or toxic environmental a future event in people whose immune systems are genetically predisposed to develop a vigorous autoimmune response against pancreatic B cell antigens. (Nolte and Karam, 2001).

2 Non-insulin dependent diabetes mellitus (NIDDM)

Type II diabetes greatly out numbers all other forms of diabetes. Patients with NIDDM are not dependant on exogenous insulin for prevention of ketonuria and are not prone to ketosis. However, they may require insulin for the correction of fasting hyperglycaemia if this cannot be achieved with the use of diet or oral agents, and they may develop ketosis under special circumstances such as severe stress precipitated by infections or trauma). The pathogenesis in type II diabetes is that the pancreas produces insulin but the body does not utilize the insulin correctly. This is primarily due to peripheral tissue insulin resistance where insulin-receptors or other intermediates in the insulin signaling pathways within body cells are insensitive to insulin and consequently glucose does not readily enter the tissue leading to hyperglycaemia .Obesity, which generally results in impaired insulin action, is a common risk factor for this type of diabetes, and most patients with type II diabetes are obese and will ultimately require multiple anti-diabetic agents to maintain adequate glycaemic control. (Manish *et al.*, 2019).

3- Gestational diabetes mellitus GDM

The gestational diabetes mellitus is defined as abnormal or impaired glucose metabolism before pregnancy and it initially appears during pregnancy. A decrease in insulin sensitivity(increase insulin resistance) is normally seen during pregnancy to spare the glucose for the fetus. GDM may lead to early embryo abnormalities or even death, pregnancy-induced hypertension syndrome, infection, polyhydramnios and premature labor. It will also affect the status of the fetus, including effects such as fetal malformation, macrosomia or stillbirth. The offspring of woman with GDM are more inclined to develop low blood sugar, respiratory distress syndrome and polycythemia. These offspring have a higher risk of developing obesity and impaired glucose tolerance and the mother with GDM is more likely to develop diabetes [mainly type 2 diabetes mellitus (DM)] later in life. (Zhang *et al.*, 2018).

Diabetes in pregnancy is associated with an imbalance of hormones, cytokines, metabolites and growth factors in the maternal and foetal compartment.

These may influence placental growth and development that are tightly regulated in time and space. The distinct effects of the diabetic environment depend on the time in gestation when diabetic insult occurs. Because of its establishment in the second half of gestation, GDM will influence placental processes in late gestation, whereas pre-gestational diabetes such as Type-I and Type-II diabetes may also affect processes in the first trimester. Altered placental function in pre-gestational diabetes may include changes in invasion ultimately leading to an enhanced risk of early pregnancy loss, growth restriction and pre-eclampsia, as well as a long-term stimulatory effect on placental growth leading to placentomegaly, which is frequently associated with diabetic pregnancies. Diabetes later in gestation affects vascularisation, storage of maternal nutrients in particular glycogen and lipids and may also enhance oxygen transfer. (Hiden and Desoye, 2010) It is noteworthy that these pregnancy pathologies related to placental dysfunction and pre-eclampsia as well as spontaneous abortions, occur more frequently when mothers are diabetic. (Merviel *et al.,* 2004)

The increasing prevalence in developing countries is related to decreasing levels of physical activity, changes in dietary patterns and increasing prevalence of obesity, the elevated levels of serum glucose, the pancreas should recompense by increasing insulin secretion by 2–2.5 times. Beta cell function deteriorates in GDM.(Rajpit *et al.*, 2013)

International Diabetes Federation (IDF) estimates, GDM affects about 14% of pregnancies worldwide, representing about 18 million births annually. (IDF, 2017) GDM which includes young age, high parity and family history; the major risk factor for the GDM is obesity making about 20% higher risk as compared to nonobese females. (Zaman *et al.*, 2013) To regulate the diagnosis of GDM, the World Health Organization (WHO) has future using a hour 75 gm OGTT with a threshold plasma glucose concentration of greater than 140 mg/dl at 120 minutes. (Balaj , 2011)

GDM is associated with upregulated hepatic glucose production (gluconeogenesis). Gluconeogenesis is increased in the fasted state, and not sufficiently suppressed in the fed sta. Catalano *et al.,*(2014) Pregnancy is a state of high metabolic activity, in which maintaining glucose homeostasis is of upmost importance.It is probable that genetic, epigenetic, and environmental factors all contribute to the development of GDM, pancreatic β-cells fail to compensate for a chronic fuel excess, leading to eventual insulin resistance, hyperglycemia, and an increased supply of glucose to the growing fetus. There is also evidence that adipose expandability, low-grade chronic inflammation, gluconeogenesis, oxidative stress, and placental factors contribute to the pathology of GDM. (Jasmine *et al.*, 2018)

The American Diabetes Association (ADA) formally classifies GDM as "diabetes first diagnosed in the second or third trimester of pregnancy ADA 2018. Placental leptin production is increased in GDM, probably as a result of placental insulin resistance, and this further contributes to hyperleptinemia. This is also thought to facilitate amino acid transport across the placenta, contributing to fetal macrosomia. Leptin is a satiety hormone secreted primarily by adipocytes in response to adequate fuel stores. It primarily acts on neurons within the arcuate nucleus of the hypothalamus to decrease appetite and increase energy spending (Pérez *et al.*, 2013).

Pregnant women GDM increases the risk of a number of short-term and long-term maternal health issues.The stress of normal pregnancy, GDM is associated with antenatal depression (Byrn *et al.*, 2015). Approximately 60% of women with a past history of GDM develop T2DM later in life (Shostrom *et al.*, 2017) the vasculature of women with a prior case of GDM is forever altered, predisposing them to cardiovascular disease (CVD). A recent study reported a 63% increased risk of CVD amongst women with a history of GDM. CVD is the number one cause of death in the world WHO, (2013–2020). In the long term, babies that are born of GDM pregnancies are at increased risk of obesity, T2DM, CVD, and associated metabolic diseases. Children born to mothers with GDM have almost double the risk of developing childhood obesity when compared with nondiabetic mothers, (Tam *et al*., 2017) In GDM, just as there is an alteration in fetal growth, the placenta is in the same intrauterine environment and therefore also undergoes alterations in its formation, structure, and function. These alterations could be related to an oxygenation deficiency in the fetus and changes in the transplacental transport of nutrients, increasing their availability to the fetus and thus causing fetal overgrowth (Prieto & Influencia 2013).

Diabetes in pregnancy is associated with concentration changes of hormones, cytokines, metabolites and growth factors in the maternal and foetal blood. These may interrupt placental growth and development GDM will effect placental processes in late gestation, whereas pre-gestational diabetes such as Type-I and Type-II diabetes may also affect processes in the first trimester. Altered placental function in pre-gestational diabetes may include changes in invasion eventually leading to an improved risk of early pregnancy loss, growth restriction and pre-eclampsia, as well as a long-term stimulatory effect on placental growth leading to placentomegaly, which is frequently associated with diabetic pregnancies. Diabetes later in gestation affects vascularization, storage of maternal nutrients in particular glycogen and lipids and may also recover oxygen transfer. (Hiden & Desoye, 2010).

GDM is defined as impaired glucose tolerance of variable severity with first onset during pregnancy. (DeSisto, *et al.,* 2014). The common mechanism in GDM is the beta cell dysfunction, due to the antagonism created by the anti-insulin hormones in pregnancy. Around nine weeks after conception, insulin is distinguished in the fetal pancreas from 16 weeks onwards. (Spranger *et al.*, 2003). The receptivity of the placenta to glucose uptake means that it is particularly sensitive to maternal hyperglycemia, and this directly contributes to increased fetal growth and macrosomia. Protein—Amino acid transport across the placenta is also an important determinant of fetal growth, normal glucose metabolism returns within 1 year postpartum. (Zhang *et al.*, 2016).

References --

Aditiawarman (2014). The role of albumin and endoplasmic reticulum in pathogenesis Preeclampsia. Changes of GRP78 and placental VEGF in preeclampsia. Pregnancy Hypertens. 4, 247 .

AL-Khurri, L.,E., Mustafa,I.,A.,M(2010) VEGF in situ mRNA expression along with different histopathological parameters of colorectal adenocarcinoma. Al-Qadisiyah Medical Journal . Volume:6 Issue: 10 pages: 38-51 .

American Academy of Pediatrics Committee on Fetus and Newborn and American College of Obstetricians and Gynecologists Committee on Obstetric Practice.(2015) Pediatrics 136 (4) 819-822 .

American Diabetes Association. Classification and Diagnosis of Diabetes: Standards of Medical Care in Diabetes—2018. Diabetes Care 2018, 41, S13–S27.

Ariadne Malamitsi-Puchner, Theodora Boutsikou, Emmanuel Economou, Angeliki Sarandakou, Evangelos Makrakis, Dimitrios Hassiakos, and George Creatsas (2005) Vascula Endothelial Growth Factor and Placenta Growth Factor in

Intrauterine Growth-Restricted Fetuses and Neonates. Mediators of Inflammation•5th, 293–297

Arsenio Spinilloa,∗, Barbara Gardellaa, Giulia Muscettolaa, Stefania Cesarib, Giacomo Fiandrinob Chryssoula Tziallac. (2019)The impact of placental massive perivillous fibrin deposition on neonatal outcome in pregnancies complicated by fetal growth restriction. Placenta J. v (87), p. 46-52.

Ashfaq, M.; Janjua, M. Z. & Channa, M. A. (2005) Effect of gestational diabetes and maternal hypertension on gross morphology of placenta. J. Ayub. Med. Coll. Abbottabad, 17(1):44-7

Baker, F.G. and Silverton, R.E. (1985). Introduction to medical laboratory technology , 6th end. Butter worths , London ., 408 pp.

Balaj V, Balaj M, Anjalakshi C, Cynthia a, Arthi T, Seshiah V. Diagnosis of GDM in Asian-Indian women. Indian J Endocrinol Metab 2011; 15(3):187-190 .

Bancroft, J.D. and Stevens, A. (1982). Theory and Practice of Histological Techniques 2nd edition Churchill living ston, Edin-Dissolve 1 gram of hematoxylin stain powder in 10 ml of absolute ethyl alcohol.

Barnwalet M, Rathi SK, Chhabra S, Nanda S (2012). Histomorphometry of umbilical cord and its vessels in pre-eclampsia as compared to normal pregnancies. NJOG.7(1):28-32.

Bastos Aires, M. & dos Santos, A. C. V. (2015) Effects of maternal diabetes on trophoblast cells. World J. 4er fv Diabetes, 6(2):338-344 .

Beck, M. (2009) How is your baby? Recalling the Apgar score's namesake. Health journal, 1-3.

.

Bhanu SP, Sankar DK, Swetha M (2016). Morphological and micrometrical changes of the placental terminal villi in normal and pregnancies complicated with gestational diabetes mellitus. J. Evid. Based Med. Healthc. ; 3(68), 3676-3680.

Blackburn, S. Prenatal Period and Placental Physiology. Maternal, Fetal & Neonatal Physiology. 4th ed. Maryland Heights, Saunders, 2013. pp.79-85.

Burton G.J. Anatomy and genesis of the placenta. In: Neill J.D., editor. Knobil and Neill's Physiology of Reproduction. third edition. Elsevier; 2006. pp. 189–243.

Byrn, M.; Penckofer, S. The relationship between gestational diabetes and antenatal depression. J. Obstet. Gynecol. Neonatal Nurs. 2015, 44, 246–255 .

Carlson, 2014). Carlson, B. M. Embriología Humana y Biología del Desarrollo. 5th ed. Ann Arbour, Elsevier, 2014.

Castejon OC, Lopez GAJ (2018). Scanning Electron Microscopy of Placental Villi Associated to Four Complications of Pregnancy. J Emerg Rare Dis. Jan;1(1):104

Castejón, O. C. & Molinaro, M. P. Madurez de las vellosidades coriales y su relación con desordenes hipertensivos en casos de desprendimiento prematuro grave de placenta normoinserta. Rev. Fac. Cienc. Salud Univ. Carabobo, 8(3):17-26, 2004.

Catalano, P.M. Trying to understand gestational diabetes. Diabet. Med. 2014, 31, 273–281.

Chen D. B., Zheng J. (2014). Regulation of placental angiogenesis. Microcirculation 21, 15–25 .

Cianni GD, Miccoli R, Volpe L, Lencioni C, Del Prato S(2003). Intermediate metabolism in normal pregnancy and in gestational diabetes. Diabetes Metab Res Rev. 2003;19:259–70 .

Clark, M. Lin, M. Tawhai, R. Saghian, and J. L. James. (2015) Multiscale modelling of the feto–placental vasculature 6; 5 .(2)

Debashish Bhattacharjee, Santosh Kumar Mondal, Pratima Garain,1 Palash Mandal,2 Rudra Narayan Ray, and Goutam Dey. (2017) Histopathological study with immunohistochemical expression of vascular endothelial growth factor in placentas of hyperglycemic and diabetic women. J Lab Physicians. 9(4): 227–233.

Dellinger MT, Brekken RA. (2011) Phosphorylation of Akt and ERK1/2 is required for VEGF-A/VEGFR2-induced proliferation and migration of lymphatic endothelium. PLoS One. 6 .(12)

Demir R, Kayisli UA, Cayli S, Huppertz B.(2006) Sequential steps during vasculogenesis and angiogenesis in the very early human placenta. Placenta. ;27:535–9 .

Demir R, Kayisli UA, Seval Y, Celik-Ozenci C, Korgun ET, Demir-Weusten AY(2004). Sequential expression of VEGF and its receptors in human placental villi during very early pregnancy: Differences between placental vasculogenesis and angiogenesis. Placenta. 2004;25:560–7

DeSisto CL, Kim SY, Sharma AJ. Prevalence Estimates of Gestational Diabetes Mellitus in the United States, Pregnancy Risk Assessment Monitoring System (PRAMS), 2007-2010. Prev Chronic Dis 2014;11:130415.

Desoye G, Hauguel-de Mouzon S. The human placenta in gestational diabetes mellitus. The insulin and cytokine network. Diabetes Care 2007; 30 (Suppl 2): S120–S126 .

Dockery, P., Bermingham, J., and Jenkins, D. (2000) Structure–function relations in the human placenta. Biochemical Society Transactions (2000), Volume 28, part2,204-207 .

Donnini S, Ztche M, and Morbidelli L., (2004). Molecular Mechanisms of VEGF-Induced Angiogenesis. VEFG and Cancer.chapter three.edited by Judith H.Harmy

El-Sisy NA.(1999). Imunohistochemical detection of P53 in an amelobleastoma. J.of oral pathology; 5: 478-489.

Ferrara N., 2004. Vascular endothelial growth factor as a target for anticancer therapy. The Oncologist, 9: 2-10 .

Forozan Milani1 ID , Seyedeh Hajar Sharami1, Ehsan Kazemnejad Lili2, Fatemeh Ebrahimi1* ID , SeyedehFatemeh Dalil Heirati1(2019) .Association Between Umbilical Cord Coiling Index and Prenatal Outcomes international Journal of Women's Health and Reproduction Sciences Vol. 7, No. 1, 1th, 85–91.

Gauster M, Desoye G, Totsch M, Hiden U. The placenta and gestational diabetes mellitus. Curr Diab Rep. 2012;12(1):16–23.

Georgiadis L., Keski-Nisula L., Harju M. (2014) Umbilical cord length in singleton gestations: a finnish population-based retrospective register study. Placenta 35, 275–280.

Gos M., Bomba-Opon D. (2015). Placental pathologic changes in gestational diabetes mellitus. Neuro Endocrinol. Lett. 36, 101–10

Guodong Fu, Jelena Brkić, Heyam Hayder, and Chun Peng*(2013).MicroRNAs in Human Placental Development and Pregnancy Complications. Int J Mol Sci. 8; 14(3): 5519–5544

Gutiérrez J., Droppelmann C. A., Salsoso R., Westermeier F., Toledo F., Salomon C., et al. . (2016). A hypothesis for the role of RECK in angiogenesis. Curr. Vasc. Pharmacol. 14, 106–115 .

Hiden U, Desoye G. The Placenta in a Diabetic Pregnancy 2010. J. Reproduktionsmed. Endokrinol 7 (1), 27-33.

Hodges GM, Car KE (1983). Biomedical research applications of scanning electron microscopy. Vol 3. London: Academic Press, 1983.

Hyder SM, Huang JC, Nawaz Z, (2000). Regulation of vascular endothelial growth factor expression by estrogens and progestins. Environ Health Perspect. 108(suppl 5):785–790

International Diabetes Federation. IDF Diabetes Atlas, 8th ed.; IDF: Brussels, Belgium, 2017 .

Jain A, Ranjan R, Jha K. Histomorphometry of umbilical cord in gestational diabetes mellitus. Medical Science. 2014;6(21):71-73.

Jarmuzek P., Wiel Georgiadis L., Keski-Nisula L., Harju M. (2014). Umbilical cord length in singleton gestations: a finnish population-based retrospective register study. Placenta 35, 275–280 .

Jarmuzek P., Wielgos M., Bomba-Opon D. (2015). Placental pathologic changes in gestational diabetes mellitus. Neuro Endocrinol. Lett. 36, 101–10

Jasmine F Plows 1 , Joanna L Stanley 2, Philip N Baker 3, Clare M Reynolds 2 and Mark H.(2012). The Pathophysiology of Gestational Diabetes Mellitus . Int. J. Mol. Sci. 2018, 19, 3342 5 of 21

Jauniaux E., Watson A. L., Hempstock J., Bao Y. P., Skepper J. N., Burton G. J. (2000). Onset of maternal arterial blood flow and placental oxidative stress. A possible factor in human early pregnancy failure. Am. J. Pathol. 157, 2111–2122.

Jia,p.L., Brkićb,J.,Liua,M.,Chun ,F.and Yan-LingWanga (2013)Placental trophoblast cell differentiation: Physiological regulation and pathological relevance to preeclampsia .Molecular Aspects of Medicine.Volume 34, Issue 5, Pages 981-1023.

.

Kaufmann, P. and Burton, G. (1994) Anatomy and Genesis of the Placenta, in The Physiology Of Reproduction (Knobil, E. and Neill, J. D., eds.), pp. 441–484, Raven Press, New York

Kelly E. Johnson, Traci A. Wilgus (2014). Vascular Endothelial Growth Factor and Angiogenesis in the Regulation of Cutaneous Wound Repair. 1; 3(10): 647–661.

Khan R, Ali K, Khan Z.(2013) Socio-demographic risk factors of Gestational Diabetes Mellitus. Pak J Med Sci. 29(3):843-46
Kiernan JA (2008) Histological and Histochemical Methods: Theory and Practice. 4th ed. Bloxham, UK: Scion.

Kiernan JA (2008) Histological and Histochemical Methods: Theory and Practice. 4th ed. Bloxham, UK: Scion.

Kingdom J, Huppertz B, Seaward G, Kaufmann P. (2000) Development of the placental villous tree and its consequences for fetal growth. Eur J Obstet Gynecol Reprod Biol. 92:35–43

Koch S, Claesson-Welsh L. (2012) Signal transduction by vascular endothelial growth factor receptors. Cold Spring Harb Perspect Med. 2 :(7)

Kociszewska,k.,Czekaj,p. (2017). New Insight into Progesterone-dependent Signalization.Pharmaceutical Sciences Journal, 4, 11-22 .

Kulkarni, M.L., Matadh, S.P., Ashok, C., Pradeep N., Avinash T. and Kulkarni A.M. (2007) Absence of Wharton's jelly around the umbilical arteries. Indian Journal of Pediatrics, 74 (8): 787-789

Kumar, V.; Cotran, S. & Robin, S. L. Basic Pathology. 6th ed. Pennsylvania, W. B. Saunders, 2000.

Kumazaki K, Nakayama M, Suehara N, Wada Y. (2002) Expression of vascular endothelial growth factor, placental growth factor, and their receptors Flt-1 and KDR in human placenta under pathologic conditions. Hum Pathl. 33: 1069–77 .

Lassance L., Miedl H., Absenger M., Diaz-Perez F., Lang U., Desoye G., et al. . (2013). Hyperinsulinemia stimulates angiogenesis of human fetoplacental endothelial cells: a possible role of insulin in placental hypervascularization in diabetes mellitus. J. Clin. Endocrinol. Metab. 98, E1438–E1447.

Li, J.; Song, L.; Zhou, L.; Wu, J.; Sheng, C.; Chen, H.; Liu, Y.; Gao, S.; Huang, W. (2015) .A MicroRNA Signature in Gestational Diabetes Mellitus Associated with Risk of Macrosomia. Cell. Physiol. Biochem. Int. J.Exp. Cell. Physiol. Biochem. Pharmacol. 37, 243–252.

Linda, M. (2018). Ernst Maternal vascular malperfusion of the placental bed J.placenta pathology; 126:551-560

Linde LE, Rasmussen S, Kessler J, Ebbing C (2018) Extreme umbilical cord lengths, cord knot and entanglement: Risk factors and risk of adverse outcomes, a population-based study. PLoS ONE 13(3)

Luis Sobrevia,1,2,3,* Rocío Salsoso,1,3 Bárbara Fuenzalida,1 Eric Barros,1 Lilian Toledo,1 Luis Silva,1 Carolina Pizarro,1 Mario Subiabre,1 Roberto Villalobos,1 Joaquín Araos,1 Fernando Toledo,4 Marcelo González,5,6 Jaime Gutiérrez,1,7 Marcelo Farías,1 Delia I. Chiarello,1 Fabián Pardo,1 and Andrea Leiva1.(2016)

Insulin Is a Key Modulator of Fetoplacental Endothelium Metabolic Disturbances in Gestational Diabetes Mellitus. Front Physiol. 7: 119

M Yousuf Sarwar, Nilesh Kumar, Nawal Kishor Pandey (2013). Servation on vascular pattern of chorionic blood vessels of placenta. J OB. 10 v(2) issue44 Page: 8650-865

Madazli R, Tuten A, Calay Z, Uzun H, Uludag S, Ocak V.(2008) The incidence of placental abnormalities, maternal and cord plasma malondialdehyde and vascular endothelial growth factor levels in women with gestational diabetes mellitus and nondiabetic controls. Gynecol Obstet Invest.; 65(4):227–32 .

Manisha Bisht, D.C. Dhasmana, and S.S. Bist.(2010) Angiogenesis: Future of pharmacological modulation Indian J Pharmacol. 42(1): 2–8 .

Manish Kumar Maurya, Rajeev Kumar Varma , Ishwar Chandra chaurasia, Ravikant Vishwakarma ,Nitin Yadav(2019). A review Literature on science of Diabetes mellitus. IJ RAR ,v: 6, issue 2: 902

Mirbod P.(2018) Analytical model of the feto-placental vascular system: consideration of placental oxygen transport. R. Soc. open sci.5: 180219

Mayhew TM. Fetoplacental angiogenesis during gestation is biphasic, longitudinal and occurs by proliferation and remodelling of vascular endothelial cells. Placenta. 2002;23:742–50 .

Mitrović M, Stojić S, Tešić DS (2014). The impact of diabetes mellitus on the course and outcome of pregnancy during a 5-year follow-up. Military-medical and pharmaceutical review ;71(10):907–914.

Moffett, Susan E. Hiby, and Andrew M. Sharkey (2015) The role of the maternal immune system in the regulation of human birthweight 5; 370(1663).

Nagy JA, Dvorak AM, Dvorak H. (2003) VEGF-A(164/165) and PlGF: roles in angiogenesis and arteriogenesis. Trends Cardiovasc Med. 13(5):169–75 .

Nagy, B.; Szekeres-Barthó, J.; Kovács, G.L.; Sulyok, E.; Farkas, B.; Várnagy, Á.; Vértes, V.; Kovács, K.; Bódis, J. Key to Life: Physiological Role and Clinical Implications of Progesterone. Int. J. Mol. Sci. 2021, 22,

Oh M. J., Zhang C., LeMaster E., Adamos C., Berdyshev E., Bogachkov Y., et al. . (2016). Oxidized-LDL signals through Rho-GTPase to induce endothelial cell stiffening and promote capillary formation. J. Lipid Res. 10.1194/jlr.M062539 .

Olivar Clemente Castejón Sandoval y Angela Josmar López González(2013). A light and Scanning Electrone Microscopy Study of Placental Villi Associated With Obesity and Htpertention Rev Electron Biomed / Electron J Biomed 2013;2:29-36.

Oratz, S. (2014). The Hormones of the Placenta. The Science Journal of the Lander College of Arts and. Sciences, 8(1).

PanelK.Orendia1V.Kivityb1M.SammarbcY.GrimpelbR.GonendH.MeiribE.Lubzense B.Huppertza(2011) .Placental and trophoblastic in vitro models to study preventive and therapeutic agents for preeclampsia. Volume 32, Supplement 1, Pages S49-S54

Parham P, Moffett A. 2013. Variable NK cell receptors and their MHC class I ligands in immunity, reproduction and human evolution. Nat. Rev. Immunol. 13, 133–144.

Pérez-Pérez, A.; Maymó, J.L.; Gambino, Y.P.; Guadix, P.; Dueñas, J.L.; Varone, C.L.; Sánchez-Margalet, V. Activated translation signaling in placenta from pregnant women with gestational diabetes mellitus: Possible role of leptin. Horm. Metab. Res. 2013, 45, 436–442..

Peter Kelehan and Paul Downey. (2018) Villous Oedema. In (Pathology of the Placenta. Springer com.) pp 153-155 Srinivasan, A. P.; Omprakash, B. O. & Lavanya, K.; Subbulakshmi Murugesan, P. & Kandaswamy, S. (2014) A prospective study of villous capillary lesions in complicated pregnancies. J. Pregnancy, Nov 24. 10.1155

Pietro L, Daher S, Rudge MV, Calderon IM, Damasceno DC, Sinzato YK, Bandeira C, Bevilacqua E. (2010) Vascular endothelial growth factor (VEGF) and VEGF-receptor expression in placenta of hyperglycemic pregnant women. Placenta. 31(9):770–80.

Pijnenborg, L. Vercruysse, M. Hanssens (2006). The uterine spiral arteries in human pregnancy: facts and controversies. Placenta 27 939-958 .

Predanic M (2009). Sonographic assessment of the umbilical cord. Donald School J Ultrasound Obstet Gynecol. 3(2):48-57.

Prieto Gómez, R.; Matamala, F. & Rojas, M. (2008)Características morfológicas y morfométricas de la placenta de término, en recién nacidos pequeños para la edad gestacional (PEG) en la ciudad de Temuco-Chile. Int. J. Morphol., 26(3):615-21

Prieto Gómez, R.; Smok, C. & Rojas, M (2011). Experiencias de blog: Placenta comparada. Int. J. Morphol., 29(2):432-5.

Prieto Sanchez, T. (2013). Influencia de la Diabetes Mellitus Gestacional en Parámetros Antropométricos y Bioquímicos Materno-Fetales y en la Transferencia Placentaria de Ácidos Grasos. Tesis doctoral. Murcia, Universidad de Murcia.

Qian Meng, Li Shao, Xiucui Luo, Yingping Mu, Wen Xu, Chao Gao, Li Gao, Jiayin Liu, Yug ui Cui(2015). "Ultrastructure of Placenta of Gravidas with Gestational Diabetes Mellitus", Obstetrics and Gynecology International, vol . 9 pages Endocrinol. Sep 20, 14: 61

Rajpit R, Yadev Y, Navida S, Rajput M (2013). Prevalence of Gestational diabetes mellit us and associated risk factors at a tertiary care hospital in Haryana. Indian J Med Res 2013; 137(4):728-733 .

Rani A, Wadhwani N, Chrean p., Joshi,S., (2016) Altered developments and function of the placenta . Wiley review .,Development Biology.

Rebecca,B.(2005). Proliferation of villous trophoblastof human placentain normal and abnormal pregnancy virchows Arch. B. cell Pathol. Vol. 60:pp.365-372.

Reis FM1, D'Antona D, Petraglia F.(2002). Predictive value of hormone measurements in maternal and fetal complications of pregnancy. Endocr Rev. 2002 Apr;23(2):230-57 .

Roa, I.; Smok, C. & Prieto Gómez, R. Placenta: Anatomía e histología comparada. Int. J. Morphol., 30(4):1490-6, 2012.

Robert Amadu Ngala, Linda Ahenkorah Fondjo, Peter Gmagna, , Frank Naku Ghartey, Martin Akilla Awe (2017) Placental peptides metabolism and maternal factors as predictors of risk of gestational diabetes in pregnant women. A case-control study. PLoS One. 12(7):

Ruth Prieto Gómez ; Nicolás Ernesto Ottone2, 3 & Homero Bianchi. (2018) Morphological Features of the Human Placenta and its Free Chorionic Villi in Normal Pregnancies and those with Diabetes and and high blood pressure. Int. J. Morphol., 36(4):1183-1192.

SPathak[a]E.Hook[b]G.Hackett[a]E.Murdoch[c]N.J.Sebire[d]F.Jessop[b]C.Lees .(2010) Cord coiling, umbilical cord insertion and placental shape in an unselected cohort delivering at term: Relationship with common obstetric outcomes. Volume 31, Issue 11, November 2010, Pages 963-968.

.

Saddler TW (2004). Placenta and fetal membranes. In: Langman's medical embryology. Lippincott Williams & Wilkins .91-111.

Saddler.T.W..1995. Langmans medical embryology. William & Wilkins 7th .page:108-110

Saghian R,Bogles G, James J.,Clark R.(2019) Establishments of maternal blood supply .Royal Society Journal .16,9,issue 5.

Saundar M. (2009) Transplacental transport of nanomaterials.Biology,Medicine .

Sandra V. Ashton, Guy St. J. Whitley, Philip R. Dash, Mark Wareing, Ian P. Crocker, Philip N. Baker, Judith E. Cartwright (2000). Uterine Spiral Artery Remodeling Involves Endothelial Apoptosis Induced by Extravillous Trophoblasts Through Fas/FasL Interactions. (Biochemical Society Transactions (2000), Volume 28, part 2.

Seema Valsalan Ennazhiyili, PK Ramakrishnan2, VR Akshara3, KS Premlal4, S Chitra5, W Benjamin6, Saranya Nagalingam7. (2019) Effects of Gestational Diabetes Mellitus on Umbilical Cord. Journal of Clinical and Diagnostic Research. Jul, Vol-13:(7)

Seo J. H., Yu J. H., Suh H., Kim M. S., Cho S. R. (2013). Fibroblast growth factor-2 induced by enriched environment enhances angiogenesis and motor function in chronic hypoxic-ischemic brain injury. PLoS ONE 8:e74405.

Sharmila Bhanu P, Devi Sankar, Swetha M, Sujatha Kiran (2016). Placental terminal villi in normal and pregnancy complicated with gestational diabetes mellitus. J.Evid.Based Med Health Vol 3(68) .3676-3680.

Shibuya M. (2013) Vascular endothelial growth factor and its receptor system: physiological functions in angiogenesis and pathological roles in various diseases. J Biochem. 153(1):13–9 .

Shostrom, D.C.V.; Sun, Y.; Oleson, J.J.; Snetselaar, L.G.; Bao, W(2017). History of Gestational Diabetes Mellitus in Relation to Cardiovascular Disease and Cardiovascular RiskFactors in US Women. Front. Endocrinol. 8, 144.

Silva J.F., Serakides R (2016). Intrauterine trophoblast migration: A comparative view of humans and rodents. Cell Adh. Migr.10:88–110.

Spranger J, Kroke A, Mohlig M, Bergmann MM, Ristow M, Boeing H, (203). Adiponectin and protection against type 2 diabetes mellitus. Lancet. 2003; 361:226-8 .

Sudha R, Sivakumar V, Christilda FJ (2012). Study of shape of placental weight in normal and complicated pregnancies. Nat J Basic Med Sci ;2(4):307-311.

Sujatha M. S., Madhana S.*, Shylaja P., Priyanka S. (2019) Role of sex hormone binding globulin as the early predictor for gestational diabetes mellitus. Int J Reprod Contracept Obstet Gynecol. Volume 8 · Issue 3 Page 968.

Sun L, Jin Z, Teng W, Chi X, Zhang Y, Ai W and Wang P (2013): SHBG in GDM maternal serum, placental tissues and umbilical cord serum expression changes and its significance. Diabetes Res Clin Pract. 99:168–173.

Tam, W.H.; Ma, R.C.W.; Ozaki, R.; Li, A.M.; Chan, M.H.M.; Yuen, L.Y.; Lao, T.T.H.; Yang, X.; Ho, C.S.; Tutino, G.E.; (2017). In Utero Exposure to Maternal Hyperglycemia Increases Childhood Cardiometabolic Risk in Offspring. Diabetes Care , 40, 679–686 .

Tennant, P. W.; Glinianaia, S. V.; Bilous, R. W.; Rankin, J. & Bell, R. (2014) Preexisting diabetes, maternal glycated haemoglobin, and the risks of fetal and infant death: a population-based study. Diabetologia, 57(2):285- 94.5

TroncosoF, Acurio J, Herlitz K, Aguayo C, Bertoglia P, Guzman-Gutierrez E. (2017) Gestational diabetes mellitus is associated with increased pro-migratory activation of vascular endothelialgrowth factor receptor 2 and reduced expressionof vascular endothelial growth factor receptor 1. PLoS ONE 12(8).

Uzan S. 2004 Pathophysiology of preeclampsia: links with implantation disorders. Eur J Obstet Gynecol Reprod Biol; 115: 134–147.

VERMAM, R.; PRASAD, R.; MISHRA, S. & KAUL, J. M. (2012) Vascular pattern of chorionic blood vessels of placenta and its correlation with the birth weight of neonate. Int. J. Morphol., 30(3):952-955.

World Health Organization (WHO). Global Action Plan for the Prevention and Control of NCDs 2013–2020; WHO: Geneva, Switzerland, 2013 .

Yao Ye, Aurelia Vattai, Xi Zhang, Junyan Zhu, Christian J. Thaler, Sven Mahner, Udo Jeschke,* and Viktoria von Schönfeldt. (2017) Role of Plasminogen Activator Inhibitor Type 1 in Pathologies of Female Reproductive Diseases. Int J Mol Sci. Aug; 18(8): 1651 .